CANC

fallacies and some reassuring facts

Cancer Prevention

FALLACIES AND SOME REASSURING FACTS

by Cyril Scott

ATHENE PUBLISHING CO. LTD.
Wellingborough, Northamptonshire

First published 1968
Second Impression 1970
Third Impression 1971
Fourth Impression 1974
Fifth Impression 1976
Sixth Impression 1978
Seventh Impression 1980

ISBN 0 7225 0260 5

Made and Printed in Great Britain by Weatherby Woolnough Ltd., Wellingborough Northants, England

Contents

Introduction

There is no denying that about some important problems in life the truth can only be discovered when several branches of knowledge are brought into alignment—in other words, when knowledge has been pooled and shared. But unfortunately where the problem of cancer is concerned, there has been a noticeable reluctance to do this very necessary thing. The result is that on the one hand we have in the different countries the various self-regarding orthodox medical organisations with their views and pronouncements about the dreaded disease, and on the other hand the exponents of the unorthodox systems of therapeutics who to a large extent disagree with those views. In consequence the general public, which largely and dutifully pins its faith to what is orthodox, has acquired only a one-sided conception of the whole matter, and thus it is left to unbiased writers who have studied it from every angle to adjust the balance by presenting all the available facts.

There are also the fallacies to be considered which tend to create *fear*, as they obviously do, in the minds of numerous people, and should for that reason among others be rectified as far as possible. I write with sympathy for my fellows, having suffered when a very young and neurasthenic man from the fear of cancer myself. Incidentally, that fear vanished in a very short time as did some other manifestations of general unfitness as soon as I adjusted my mode of living and feeding to one more in accordance with naturopathic principles: which, however, is not to imply that the following pages constitute a treatise on naturopathy.

This much shorter book, as also my earlier and larger one on the same subject, is the outcome of having for over fifty years in my spare time investigated the claims and testimonies of those systems of healing, which medical Orthodoxy for the most part has been pleased to ignore as incompatible with its own beliefs. Nor is that all; for the devotees of Orthodoxy—allowing as we shall see for a good many exceptions—have likewise ignored or discountenanced the discoveries and achievements of doctors even with orthodox qualifications; namely ones who have cured cancer without the usual recourse to surgery, ray-therapy or both these drastic means. Therefore it is only just and right that those discoveries and achievements should be more widely made known to the public at large.

And here at the outset I wish to stress that any critical references in this book to the Orthodox fraternity are made in no hostile spirit; hundreds of whose members, I doubt not for a moment are other than selfless and altruistic men, several of whom I may add, having in their lifetimes been among my valued personal friends. But so likewise have been practitioners of the less advertised therapies; homoeopaths, osteopaths, naturopaths, biochemists of the Schuessler system, and medical herbalists. Moreover I have seen proof of long-standing and painful complaints cured by such practitioners after orthodox treatments had completely failed . . . Yet in mentioning the cure of these chronic afflictions, no denial is implied as to the considerable achievements of Orthodox medicine in reducing both the gravity and high mortality rate of so many of our erstwhile acute diseases. But with such, this book is not concerned.

I grant it may be an inexactitude to speak of preventing in a person or number of persons any disease unless one is first sure that otherwise it would certainly occur. But there are other considerations, *viz.*, ones relating to the general health which, as the reader will come to see, have an important bearing on our subject.

THE PRESENT-DAY BELIEF

Generally speaking it would be reasonably safe to say that the prevalent notion about cancer is that despite years and years of research, its root cause still remains a mystery; and although more commonly occurring in elderly people, nowadays it may even be found in quite young ones and in children also, mostly in the form of leukaemia, said to be a type of cancer of the blood.

This verdict which the general public largely accepts, is conducive to *fear*, because it even carries implication that the cause or causes of the dreaded disease being unknown, it may not be even preventible. Yet, the regrettable and, alas, all too obvious fact is that only by constantly reminding us of the disease, and thus unavoidably fostering that fear, can the donations be acquired to finance cancer research, grown to costly proportions since it became an institution. Nor has that fear been lessened by the publicised advice that one should undergo regular periodic tests to discover if there be any incipient signs of the affliction. If there be no such sign, then according to research conclusions, it means that the body of the person examined possesses that mysterious "something" which stated in the simplest words prevents the occurrence of malignancy.

And more definitely explicit than that, it would

seem, the orthodox cancer research ring is not prepared to be, either because unable or unwishful—at least, judging from what a distinguished lady scientist (since deceased) confided to me erewhile. She told me that she had turned down a request to associate herself with a large research establishment because of a ruling that she must only give out that her research work was leading to an important discovery, but she must *not* disclose the conclusion at which she had arrived. Yet whatever construction the reader may think to put on this strange stipulation, there remains the noticeable fact that when from time to time a new theory has been announced, the statement has nearly always been followed by a warning that more research would be needed before it could be proved.

This of course has meant and still means delay in solving the cancer problem, at any rate as far as the public is concerned. But that is not to say that a number of individual physicians have failed to solve it to the extent of being able to cure their patients; as will be seen from the following paragraphs.

PART I

SOME FACTS, FALLACIES AND FRUSTRATIONS

Homoeopathic Achievements

Writing in 1929, Dr. A. H. Grimmer, M.D., of U.S.A., said: "The curing of cancer cases by homoeopathic remedies is nothing new or strange. . . . In the past four years I have treated two hundred and twenty-five cases of proven cancer, of various forms and in all stages of the disease. At this time (1929) one hundred and seventy-five are still living, many of them entirely well and free of all cancer symptoms, only one of this group shows indications of an early demise. All of those who failed to respond to the homoeopathic treatment had been treated, surgically or with X-ray and radium in material doses" (*The Homoeopathic Recorder*). It is important to mention here that the doctor stressed the necessity of putting the patients on an entirely vegetarian and fruitarian diet; a statement which becomes highly significant if noted in conjunction with what will be revealed in due course. Meanwhile it should be especially noted that Dr. Grimmer began his article with a reference to the fact that the *curing* (my italics) of cancer cases by homoeopathic remedies was neither new or strange; the obvious implication being that homoeopaths had already been able to cure the disease long before 1929.

Even so, impressive though the cures thus effected may be, the homoeopathic method, one cannot deny, does give its doctors more trouble and time than does the orthodox system of treating disease as largely practised today compared with how it used to be practised.

In the old days individual doctors used to make up their prescriptions to cure, as they hoped, each individual patient's complaints. But nowadays things are different. From the bewildering assortment of drugs such as tranquillizers, pain-killers, pep-pills, patent medicines and what-not sold by the drug manufacturers, the general habit is for the doctors simply to select one or other from this vast array calculated to cure or alleviate given ailments, even though these doctors have at first little else to go on but the manufacturers' word for it. That word may be given in all good faith; nevertheless there is no denying that whatever the selected drug may be, it does not allow for the idiosyncracies of individual patients; yet as wise homoeopathic physicians have pointed out, this is of the utmost importance, and so is always taken into account by competent homoeopaths.

And why? For the simple and obvious reason that the name of a disease is far from always an indication of its cause, which may be and often is a psychological or emotional one.

It is instructive to note the following case: a man afflicted with diabetes consulted a homoeopath of my acquaintance, who proceeded to give him the usually indicated medicaments, but with no remedial effect. Finally he discovered after much questioning that his patient had some years previously suffered a great grief. He then gave him the homoeopathic remedy for grief—and that cured the diabetes.

This case is only one among many which tends to prove that although the names of some commonly known disorders can often be a time-saving guide to their treatment by orthodox means, it is not always a reliable guide, as already implied and as numerous other cases have shown. For according to homoeopaths, a number of chronic diseases may all too often be due to some acute ones having been *suppressed* by drugs instead of factually cured by them. For instance, how often does one hear a person say, "I've never felt quite the same since I had that illness some time ago." This means that the toxins have still remained in the system and affected the general health, which as every homoeopath knows, cannot be expected to improve until those toxins have been got rid of by the appropriate treatment.

Naturally, in a country possessing a National Health Service, a doctor's time is a consideration to be reckoned with, and may account for the decrease in the number of homoeopathic practitioners during the last decades, in that the majority of medical students prefer to study the orthodox system; one result being that nowadays hundreds of people are quite ignorant of what homoeopathy in truth is, and of its value as a method of curing human ills, not excluding numerous cases of cancer, as already mentioned. Yet although all this may remind us how reputations in medical treatments are apt to arise and diminish, no more need here be said about that aspect of our thesis: therefore let us deal with its other aspects.

Two Differing Contentions

In the early part of this century, two English doctors aroused the disapproval of their conventional confreres by declaring that cancer could never occur in a perfectly healthy body. But actually true though this may be, it conflicts with the current belief that even "perfect health" gives no real protection against the disease; for if it did, one might ask, how is it that a number of men and women who for years have seemingly enjoyed excellent health should none the less in the end develop malignant symptoms without any apparent reason?

And yet this fact is not puzzling to naturopaths or exponents of the (Schuessler) biochemic system of medicine who hold that the prerequisite to perfect health *and* its maintenance depends on the presence in the body of certain natural elements, without which permanent fitness and well-being cannot be assured. If the organism be lacking to any extent in these so-termed tissue-salts, or in the course of time it becomes depleted of them or there is an imbalance of them, then one or other of the well-known chronic diseases is likely to be the result. This is not to say that a surprising number of people reach old age despite a perpetually ailing body; but it is to say according to the biochemists that if the body of a person lacks those particular salts essential to preserve the normal, healthy condition of the cells, then a morbid growth is apt to occur; for which, as is commonly known, the orthodox, conventional treatment is recourse to the surgeon's knife. Nevertheless, the following considerations cannot be ignored.

Surgery: Its Limitations

Now no reasonable being will dispute that—all honour to clever surgeons—surgery has made spectacular strides during the last few decades. And yet it is unreasonable to suppose that a disease can be permanently cured merely by cutting away its *effect* instead of removing its cause. Granted that a cancerous growth occurs when a number of cells in the body run riot, so to say, and proliferate, yet that does not explain *why* they should proliferate, and so we are still left in ignorance of the prime cause of the disease. It is no more scientific to cut out a growth than it is to cut off the big toe of a person who has gout in it! But in saying this is not to deny of course that when a tumour has reached endangering proportions and impinges on some vital organ, surgery may be the only means of prolonging life.

On the other hand it is instructive to note that some women who have had breast cancers over a number of years and refused to allow their excision, have none the less lived with them without pain and discomfort well into old age. The emphasis here is on the refusal to let those growths be touched by the knife.

It should also be emphasised that many doctors have firmly maintained that the "fashionable" recourse to surgery as the first thing to be thought of when confronted with a cancer case, is both non-curative and definitely harmful. To quote one doctor, though many others with the same conviction could be cited were it not my object to avoid increasing the size of this book: "The knife is a delusive hope. It merely terrifies, and poor wretches are mutilated." He goes on to point out that if these unfortunates survive, and are not warned to reform their bad feeding habits, then "Nature will revolt, and cause further development of the cancer disease" (Dr. R. Mallet). The word "bad" in this citation does not necessarily imply "vicious" but, as we shall enlarge upon later, a diet lacking in an adequate proportion of those elements essential to good health.

Should this observation seem somewhat trite on the surface, it is not so in the light of the collected evidence hereinafter to be submitted.

The Radium "Fashion"

Elderly people with long memories may recall how the medical world was stirred to its depths when X-rays and radium were first discovered, and how the doctors and so-called cancer experts, being at a complete loss how to cope with inoperable cases, at once grasped at the supposition that these mysterious elements could be used as a means of curing cancer itself.

Nevertheless, as Dr. F. W. Forbes Ross subsequently wrote in his highly significant and enlightening book *Cancer*, "the first trial of X-rays as a treatment for cancer was the blindest of blind leaps in the dark by even the most orthodox." Which however, as he further remarked, did not prevent it from becoming the "fashion." And thus it remained for a number of years as the accepted treatment, though in some cases the cobalt ray—latterly pronounced to be highly dangerous —was substituted. Anyhow, early in 1967, it was announced that certain doctors would soon be giving cancer patients a new form of treatment which promised to be an improvement on the conventional radio-therapy, even for combating advanced tumours.

Yet however effective in some cases this method may turn out to be, its object none the less is to induce a quicker disintegration of already formed cancerous tissues (for which purpose of course a certain kind of radiation instrument is needed) whereas surely the ideal therapy would be one with the potential to normalize those tissues instead of destroying them, and which on medical advice could simply be taken through the mouth. Indeed, according to a report to hand, such a type of treatment has already been found. In an announcement to that effect it was stated that by an extraordinary accident a team of British doctors had discovered a fungus containing some mysterious element of such effective potency as to cause even advanced tumours to disappear in the most remarkable way. Thus, cases thought to be hopeless got cured, thanks to the fungus, so it was found, whilst those in which the fungus had played no part did not.

Nevertheless, in case this spectacular finding should seem too much like a "major break-through in cancer research," the announcement included the usual warning that as yet it was too early to make any definite claims . . . And justly so, seeing that the said doctors themselves admitted that they still needed to discover the nature of the mysterious element in the fungus, and why it should have such astonishingly curative effects.

What the fate of this treatment will eventually become is not easy to predict, because where cancer is concerned, the effectiveness of a particular therapy does not ensure that it will be generally accepted and applied; since the discarding of a long established method with its costly equipment is a very formidable economic consideration, and one which might even account for its continued use despite some of the disadvantages it may possess.

As to the disadvantages of ray-therapy—at any rate in the form it was used for many years—there is this to be said. At the International Cancer Congress in Tokyo (1966) Dr. Richard Doll, Director of Britain's Medical Research Council's statistical unit stated that patients who had been treated with X-rays were more prone to leukaemia (cancer of the blood) than those not likewise treated. This observation tends to bear out what many distinguished doctors in several countries have for long maintained; *viz.* that ray-therapy does not remove the *cause* of the disease, and moreover lowers the body's resistance to it, which resistance is so important for the effecting of a permanent cure.

In any case, whatever the contentions of these doctors may be, the question is, how often would ray-therapy—and surgery also—need to be considered if more people knew of the great number of cancer cases which had been cured by comparatively simple and quite painless means. But they have *not* heard of these cases; one reason being that only a small portion of the general public read therapeutical books at all, another being ... but I leave the facts to speak for themselves.

Obstacles to the Spread of Knowledge

Some years ago I asked a *bona fide* London doctor who for over thirty years had been curing malignant growths without any form of ray-treatment or surgery, why in view of that possibility, were the more drastic methods still so much in use? His answer was, "Simply because it's the vogue." His first cancer patient, I may add, was a woman of around fifty, and at over eighty, not only had she remained cured, but was in very good health. Nevertheless, when for the enlightenment of his confreres this doctor, after having written a book on his form of treatment, submitted the manuscript to a firm of medical publishers, the answer he received was that they could not venture to publish it because of the adverse effect it would have on the sales of their books on more orthodox lines.

The doctor had already been to the Ministry of Health in order to "put his cards on the table," but only to be told in effect: "Very interesting. But here we can do nothing about it."

The doctor concerned has since died—a very old man—and what he intended should never remain a secret has died with him.

The foregoing gives at least some idea of the difficulties which face even properly qualified physicians whose findings could otherwise contribute to presenting the cancer problem in a less one-sided light.

Another book which might have contributed to that desideratum was subsequently published in England; its writer being a properly qualified doctor holding Edinburgh, Glasgow and London university degrees, who had practised for many years in New Zealand. In her book she explained how she had not only cured herself of cancer, but also over a hundred of her patients by dietetic means plus a few simple remedies. But despite the impressive number of her cures, her book met with such strong disapproval from the orthodox fraternity, that finally its publishers yielding to pressure from that body, decided not to reprint it when the original edition was sold out, and hence it is no longer available. Incidentally the author was eighty when she wrote it, and in perfect health, having since her self-cure always put her principles into practice. It seems unnecessary to add that neither surgery nor ray-therapy played any part in her methods; but abstention from salt was an important factor.

Yet Another Significant Book

This volume deals with the conclusion its author, Mr. Frank Totney, a Durban research chemist, had arrived at, i.e. that the prime cause of cancer was lack of oxygen in the body. But although after the most careful investigations he wrote his book displaying considerable knowledge and clear-thinking, and although for three years he spent much time, money and trouble in trying to induce the medical associations in the various countries to consider this new light on the cancer problem, all his efforts were quite in vain.

Nor was he the only one to put forward this viewpoint. Dr. Otto Warburg, head of the Max Planck Institute of Cell Physiology, Berlin, published his own conclusion to the same effect in an American journal, but with one important difference. Whereas Dr. Warburg maintained that when once cancerous cells had been formed through oxygen starvation, the damage done could not be remedied, Mr. Totney maintained that it could; and there is much collected evidence to prove that he was right.

PART II

VARIOUS THEORIES, PRESENT AND PAST

The Germ Theory

Since research was organised as long ago as towards the end of last century, theories about cancer-causes have become so numerous, that to detail them all would fill large tomes. Nevertheless some reference should be here included to a somewhat recent announcement (1964) that germs causing cancer had been isolated in a small London hospital. This announcement followed a few years after one of the American research establishments had stated that the dreaded affliction was due to a virus. In any case, the "germ theory" is yet another one to swell the long list of previously mooted theories. But what impact it will make on the medical community remains to be seen.

Nor can one say how much that community may be impressed by a still later reported from U.S.A. 1966, and based on a discovery made by two scientists of Wisconsin.

Very briefly stated, it is that rain contains certain radio-active particles; and thus when rained-upon tobacco is used in cigarette making and then smoked, those vapourised particles inhaled might perhaps be a cause of lung cancer. The two scientists have even suggested that tobacco growers might protect their plants from rain by placing umbrellas over them. Yet the question is, would they thrive in such conditions?

Some Earlier Theories

Mention having already been made of the germ-theory, or *fact* if so it may prove to be, some earlier theories being relevant to our subject and its completeness, may also be mentioned. Some of these theories are still more or less thought to be correct, or partially so, others questionable.

Without going so far into the past as the days of the great and wise Hippocrates, who with laudable acumen maintained that cancer was a general bodily disease which eventually caused a local growth, we find, for one, the so-termed "irritation theory", which I think originated towards the end of last century, or even perhaps earlier. In any case, it was noticed that a prolonged irritation (to give but one example) set up by a jagged tooth in the mouth was apt to cause cancer of the tongue; though this theory, be it noted, failed to account for the fact that with some persons malignant growths occurred in parts of the body where there had been no irritation.

Then there is—or at any rate was—what we might call the "soot theory." In the days when methods of sweeping chimneys were very different from what they are now, it was thought that because a number of chimney-sweeps got cancer, much contact with soot must be blamed for this.

A Later Mooted Theory

And now we have that more recent theory purporting to explain the increase of the disease during the last few decades, and much to the fore of late; *viz.* the cigarette-smoking theory. But granted that it may in some cases be a contributory cause, as a prime cause it is far from convincing. For on the one hand some people get lung cancer who have never smoked in their lives, and on the other hand, thousands and thousands of men the world over have smoked without malignant consequences long before that theory attracted any attention at all; and despite their indulgence there was much less cancer then than there is today, according to reports. In any case, the reason why some researchers do not uphold that theory should now be mentioned.

Evidence from Tests made in South Africa (1964)

These tests showed the lung cancer death-rate of South African-born white men residing in *rural* districts and smoking from 1 to 20 cigarettes a day, was only about 13 per 100,000; actually little higher than that of non-smokers residing in those areas. The implication in the last few words is therefore significant. It goes to show that pure air—in other words, a healthy environment—contributes in no small measure to cancer prevention just as it does to the prevention of a number of other disorders with no mystery attached to them nowadays. It also goes to suggest why in countries where there are fewer industrial areas, there is less cancer mortality than in countries where there are more.

This all bears out what the experiments of the late Sir Walter Fergusson Hannay revealed. Sir Walter, who was a consultant physician, had devoted the last ten years of his life to cancer research, and had written articles and letters stating the result of his findings and his reason for concluding that the increase in lung cancer was due to the increase in air pollution, not basically to the cigarette habit.

Among other of his significant observations was the following: After rats and mice had been subjected for a length of time to a continuous stream of cigarette smoke, they emerged from this experiment completely unaffected. On the other hand, after these same rats and mice had been subjected in exactly the same way to diesel fumes instead of cigarette smoke, they all developed cancer nodules in their lungs.

But however revealing this test was when first made, its significance has become the greater since the discovery that the spread of the disease is not only among humans but also among dogs and cats; notably those domiciled in industrial towns wherein they roam the air-polluted streets.

Nor must it be supposed that Sir Walter had ignored the fact that in cigarette smoke there is a carcinogenic agent called benzpyrene, of which so much importance is made by the anti cigarette-smoking campaigners. But, as Lady Fergusson Hannay pointed out, Sir Walter, in view of his own findings and that of other researchers along similar lines, could not accept the cigarette theory as a substitute for the air pollution one, because the amount of benzpyrene contained in cigarette smoke is but an infinitesimal fraction as compared with the amount plus other hydrocarbons present in the condensation of diesel exhaust and thus virtually harmless. Moreover some experiments made in Russia tend to bear this out. By means of an ingenious device, scientists made it possible for a tame rabbit to smoke nine cigarettes a day; and not only did the animal enjoy the indulgence, but actually became nervy and restless if its daily quantum were reduced. This test when reported had been continued for five years without any noticeable harm to the rabbit. On the other hand, the results of some experiments subsequently made in U.S.A. on a bevy of unfortunate dogs appeared—as they were intended to do—to support the cigarette theory.

In fine; for the present we have one lot of tests aimed at proving that the cigarette habit *per se* does not primarily cause cancer, and another lot aimed at proving that in polluted air lies its main cause. And thus a bewildered public is left without a criterion to decide the matter one way or the other.

Even so, there is still this to be said; granted that the cigarette habit is not one to be encouraged, there is a noteworthy difference between just plain smokers and those who inhale; about which statistics, at any rate as reported in the papers are too vague. Yet it would be no exaggeration to say that a large percentage of people who have acquired the cigarette habit do inhale, whereas pipe smokers very seldom are so inclined. In any case, it obviously cannot be just regarded as harmless to breathe in a mixture of tobacco and paper smoke. To realise this, one need simply observe the difference in the smoke taken into the lungs from that same smoke breathed out again; a difference which can only mean that some of its denser particles have remained *in* the lungs. Hence the obviously wise thing to do is to assist nature in ridding them of that residue. Thus, if each time immediately after finishing their smokes, inhalers would fill their lungs completely by taking a deep breath of pure fresh air, and then forcibly expelling it—repeated more than once would be better—then, according to the science-of-breath exponents, the harm done to health should be much minimised.

Yet even apart from the question of smoking, it has been found that insufficient oxygenation of the blood due to shallow breathing is, almost needless to say, one of the factors which predisposes some people to pulmonary diseases, including in some cases even lung cancer.

And now to mention a much less publicised theory.

The Meat-Eating Habit

The pronouncement officially made some forty years ago denying the existence of any evidence whatever that a non-meat diet tended to prevent cancer, was an assertion which does not tally with the following considerations. In those countries where the natives live on a flesh-free diet, cancer cases among them either do not occur at all, or are so exceedingly rare that to deny any connection between feeding habits and the disease is surely unreasonable. The animals have also to be taken into account, investigation having shown that the carnivorous ones are much more liable to get tumours than the vegetarian types. As for domestic pets, dogs (which are meat eaters) are apt to get growths, cats likewise if unwisely nurtured.

And yet, however factual it is that more vegetarians, proportionately, remain free from cancer than do non-vegetarians, there is still a misinterpretation of facts to be guarded against. For although the meat-eating custom in so-called civilised countries is neither humane nor necessary to health, to declare, as do some fanatical vegetarians that the consumption of animal flesh is the prime cause of cancer is far from being a foregone conclusion, seeing that the real cause may alternatively be—as nutrition experts maintain—because (generally speaking) the meat-eating population omits to include in its daily fare a sufficiency of those natural, vital, unprocessed foods, so essential to the health of the bodily cells, and therefore to health in general . . . But this aspect of the matter need not further be enlarged upon just here.

So we pass to another theory which has received little attention, though that is no proof it is unworthy of more.

The Over-Use of Common Salt

There is a notion that because sheep love salt, it must be good for humans. And so it may if rightly used. Even so this love of salt apparently does not become a real craving with sheep unless they are grazed on poor pasture.

In any case, as students of the (Schuessler) biochemic system of medicine will know, *nat. mur.* (sodium chloride) i.e. common salt is one of the twelve chief salts normally contained in a healthy body, and essential to regulate the fluids within and round its cells by what is technically known as endosmosis. It has other functions too, making it all the more important that salt be eaten in the right way. But modern civilised mankind, generally speaking, has formed the habit of consuming this valuable mineral in a form and amount out of all proportion to its consumption of the other important salts, thereby upsetting the chemical balance of the body. Indeed this imbalance is a matter which cannot be dismissed as devoid of significance, seeing that from laboratory tests it has been found that excess of salt is the irritant cause of cancer in debilitated constitutions (Dr. Smalpage, Australia). The word "debilitated" should here be noted, in that persons with such constitutions are more apt to develop a cancer phobia than are persons with adequate health; a phobia of this kind being a variant of an anxiety complex, and hence the emotions have also to be reckoned with, including

Effects of Prolonged Worry

Yet granted that many doctors concede that in certain circumstances constant worry may cause cancer, the reason why, though offered to the medical profession by Dr. Forbes Ross as long ago as near the start of the century, still seems to be regarded as a mystery. It amounts to this, and moreover is in accordance with the biochemic system of medicine, that prolonged worry uses up too quickly the phosphate of potash in the brain and nerves; and as that particular tissue salt is the cancer-preventing one, unless it is constantly replenished by eating an adequate amount of those vital foods in which it is present, the result may be a growth, especially if the daily diet is one in which common salt and salty foods play an undue part.*

There is also the following to adduce. In a broadcast it was stated that the fear of cancer may actually *cause* cancer. Yet even should it be true in some cases,

* Procurable from Health Food Stores is a table salt which, being biochemically balanced, has none of the toxic effects of common salt, and so may healthfully be used as a condiment, and also in cooking. It is called BIOSALT (Bios Brand). And as it contains several different forms of potassium as well as some other tissue salts beneficial to health, it is useful to prevent potassium deficiency and ordinary salt excess.

such fear is only to be expected so long as the present mystery-invested concept of the disease is the one mostly placed before and accepted by the public. Nevertheless however desirable and of scientific value it would be for the mystery-aspects of the affliction to be cleared up, meanwhile the fact not given adequate publicity in the medical press is that the said mystery-aspects have proved no obstacle to the curing of hundreds of cases by methods other than those in general use.

Having already mentioned the achievements of the homoeopathic method, it now remains to give some brief data respecting a few of the non-homoeopathic ones; not only because of their important relevance in any book dealing with cancer, but because until it is more widely known that such methods have existed for many years, the fear associated with the disease is likely to persist.

PART III

CURES ACHIEVED—AND WHAT MAY BE DEDUCED FROM THEM

Cures in Germany

To begin with that remarkable naturopath, Louis Kuhne—In his Naturopathic Establishment at Leipzig, in which even leprosy was cured, the method consisted of thoroughly detoxicating the cancer patients' bodies by a special system of baths, and by putting them on a diet from which all flesh foods were strictly excluded, and also all processed ones. In short—and this is important to note—the patients were ordered to live till cured on foods exactly as provided by Mother Nature.

To cite one among many cases was that of a man with cancer of the nose. And yet solely as the result of the above-mentioned treatment, the cancer completely disappeared without even leaving a scar. Believing, as Kuhne did, that cancer was not a local but a constitutional disease, the nose itself had not been touched; a fact which goes to prove that denatured foods plus auto-intoxication are at any rate the most common cause of a cancer diathesis. And this accords with Dr. Grimmer's ruling previously mentioned that his own cancer patients should be put on a diet of fruits, vegetables, cereals and nuts—the latter presumably chopped or ground. But whereas the American doctor effected his cures by a combination of homoeopathy and diet, and Kuhne by a combination of his special baths and diet, the end results still remain highly significant.

Kuhne had some failures, as he himself was the first to admit. If very ill persons sought his help so late as to be beyond all saving, that was inevitable. Nevertheless his successes much outnumbered his failures, which makes it all the more regrettable that at least the nature-cure diet plays no part in our orthodox cancer hospitals.

Dr. Forbes Ross' Discovery

This doctor was a qualified medico of the orthodox school who practised in London, and his revealing book was published in 1912. Without going into the learned medical details and convincing arguments contained in its pages, the fact here to be noted is this: whereas most of his confreres were in the habit of putting bicarbonate of soda in their prescriptions when it seemed to be indicated, Dr. Ross put bicarbonate of potash instead. And what did he find?—that not a single one of his *regular* patients during all the years of his practice got cancer. On the other hand, with *new* patients who came to him suffering from the disease, the story was always the same. On inquiring about their eating habits, he learnt that they had been living almost entirely on the usual English deficiency diet of flesh foods, some of them tinned, vegetables, of which all the valuable salts therein had been boiled out and thrown down the sink, white bread, puddings and pastries made of white flour, and stewed fruits sweetened with white sugar. Raw fruits formed no part of the daily diet but had only been eaten occasionally by way of luxury. As for raw greenstuffs, their inclusion in the daily nourishment had been virtually nil. Moreover, in addition to salt, bicarbonate of soda was put into the water of the boiled vegetables, that having been the custom to preserve their colour.

Thus, seeing that such a diet lacked the proportion of those natural mineral salts essential to maintain good health, and in particular lacked potassium. Dr. Forbes Ross advised all the cancer patients to adopt a régime much more in accordance with naturopathic principles. In addition he prescribed in low and assiminable quantities a potassium compound, consisting of some kinds of potassium plus a little phosphate of iron. As a result, he was able to cure an impressive number of cancer cases.

It is instructive to note that the doctor maintained that herbs with which herbalists had often succeeded in curing cancer were those especially rich in potassium salts. As against that, however, some professional researchers asserted that all such herbal "cures" were quite impossible.

But these *pros* and *cons* need not detain us. What importantly stands out is the fact that Dr. Forbes Ross did cure cancer, and by painless and comparatively simple means at that. Moreover, as a result of what he revealed in his book, a company was formed which sold his formula in tablet form and achieved therewith a remarkable number of cures. (No acknowledgement was made to Dr. Forbes Ross by the company, so I was told, though maybe incorrectly.) In any event, finally a law was introduced making it illegal for any person or firm to advertise and sell any preparation purporting to cure cancer, irrespective of whether such a preparation was genuinely curative or not. Thenceforth it was only allowed to state "For potassium deficiency" on any medicament based on the Forbes

Ross formula. (I may add that the doctor maintained that such deficiency was also conducive to arthritis.)

Tribute to Dr. Forbes Ross

That potassium may be naturally radioactive is perhaps something unsuspected by many contemporary doctors. Yet the following observations are significant: Writing a letter in *Truth* after the doctor's death, Mr. Barton Scammell, M.S.C.I. (then president of the Radium Institute in Dover) when paying tribute to him and his great work, had among other things, this to say: "... The radioactive alkali, potash, is the great oxygen-attracting element in the body ... Owing to certain defects in diet and the preparation of food, the modern civilised human being suffers from 'potassium starvation,' and the increase of cancer is a corollary in this state of affairs ..." In the same letter he also explained why the administration of the attenuated solutions of the citrate and radio-phosphate of potash the late doctor had used in his treatment should cause the cancer to retrograde and finally disappear.

Dr. Forbes Ross' book went out of print in 1937. In it he had mentioned a minor yet significant fact pointing to the all-importance of potash; *viz.*, that some of his patients who had been prematurely grey, found that after taking the potassium-compound, their hair regained its original colour.

Incidentally, if cancer should really prove to be a germ-disease, then pot. phos., which according to biotherapists is nature's supreme antiseptic, might well be worthy of consideration by more doctors in view of its prophylactic possibilities. But as it is the most soluble of all the biochemic salts, it is important to remember that it is easily lost if those foods containing it are unconservatively cooked or boiled.

Cures in U.S.A.

In the history of cancer therapeutics the name of Dr. William F. Koch most certainly deserves a prominent place. By means of a subtle chemical formula he devised to detoxicate the body, combined with a strictly naturopathic diet, the cures he achieved without recourse to surgery or ray-therapy ran into hundreds and hundreds.

He originally resided in Detroit; but his successes aroused such hostility towards him there, that he subsequently moved to Brazil, where he remained to carry on his successful treatments under the protection of what is called the Christian Medical Research League. Fortunately, despite the attempts to discredit him in U.S.A., a number of doctors are applying his methods with gratifying results.

Dr. Max Gerson's Accomplishments

In those clinics with which for twenty-five years he was associated, hundreds of cancer cases, some of them even very advanced ones, were cured by his methods without recourse to surgery or ray-treatment, in which he did not believe. What he did believe, maintain and prove, was that to cure malignant growths or tumours, no matter where located in the body, it was absolutely essential to treat the entire organism so as to remove their prime cause. That treatment, revealed in his book *A Cancer Therapy,* is for the major part based on the principles, practices and philosophy of Nature Cure, by the application of which plus assiminable doses of potassium, Dr. Gerson accomplished his undeniable cures. It is instructive to note that both he and Dr. Forbes Ross had realised the value of potash in the treatment of cancer.

There must of course be many people who wonder why, despite its proven efficacy, Dr. Gerson's method has not been adopted by his orthodox confreres, and thus not introduced in orthodox hospitals. But as my chief object in writing this book is to present facts collected for more than fifty years; and not wishing to increase its size, I must leave the whys and wherefores to the reader's imagination. And now to deal with another of those facts.

The Grape Cure

In the field of natural therapeutics this cure stands out as one of the most serviceable discoveries of our century, not only because of its almost miraculous effectiveness, but also because of its simplicity, seeing that grapes being a food and not a drug, it can be self-administered without the risk of any harmful side-results.

A good many years have passed since Johanna Brandt, N.D., Ph.N., M.A., made her momentous discovery; and being a practising neuropath in Cape Town, she had ample opportunities to prove its efficacy on her numerous patients, having first proved it on herself.

The facts are significant. Her own case was that of a large malignant growth in the stomach; and although a noted surgeon had told her that the only means of prolonging her life would be an operation, this she firmly refused to have. Thereafter followed a period of great suffering, which was brought to an end after she rightly divined the wonderful properties in grapes, and by dint of living on them exclusively for six weeks, was completely and permanently cured. Nevertheless, as she pointed out in her book *The Grape Cure*, that is not to say that with every sufferer the cure takes so long; for it depends on the severity of the case.

According to Dr. Brandt, grapes are a perfect food. They are rich in potassium, iron and other important salts, and therefore are strengthening to the whole organism. Moreover—very important to note—they contain an element which purifies the blood; in short, they are the perfect food-cum-medicine; this being the reason why the Grape Cure when rightly applied, has proved unfailingly curative in such numerous and varied ailments after other treatments have been tried in vain.

Already by 1929 this unique therapy had become sufficiently known for its enlightened discoverer to have received in all, thousands of unsolicited testimonials from every part of U.S.A., Canada, Mexico, Australia, South Africa, as well as England and Ireland. The conclusion to be drawn from these facts and figures is sufficiently obvious to need no enlarging upon. Yet this must be said: those grateful persons who had been moved to send the testimonials, were ones, of course, so placed and with enough will-power to carry out Dr. Brandt's directions essential for success. For even if all else be favourable, not everybody has the strength of will to live entirely on grapes for several weeks on end, and to persist with the treatment through those phases of natural crisis when the grapes are stimulating the body to throw off its toxins, and hence the sufferer is apt to feel (*pro tem*) especially wretched and discouraged. Even so, considering that weakness of will-power usually tends to go with bodily weakness as it does with old age, what Dr. Brandt noticed in her patients during or after the treatment is highly significant. She found that their senses had become acuter, dim eyes had brightened, faded hair had taken on new gloss, feeble voices become vibrant, complexions had cleared, and even loose teeth—due to pyorrhea—had become steadily fixed in the gums and no longer needed extraction; in short the treatment had resulted in rejuvenation.*

Is Cancer Hereditary?

Whilst this question is not directly connected with the Grape Cure itself, it is indirectly so; for opinions are not all in agreement on the point, and Dr. Brandt's case is certainly suggestive. As she states in her book, she comes of a family in which there had been much cancer and of which her own mother had also died. In consequence, she goes on to suggest, "the predisposing causes in my mother's body may have been present in my own."

Yet although this confession lends some support to the hereditary theory, its implications must not be carried so far as to create the supposition that all persons born into cancer-tainted families are inevitably prone to the disease: factually, hundreds of people despite their being thus placed, do not contract it.

* *The Grape Cure,* by Johanna Brandt, The Order of Harmony, South Africa.

A Logical Inference

The successful treatments previously outlined, having shown the important part which the consumption of natural, vital aliments played in them where the curing of cancer was concerned, is it unreasonable to accept, as do naturopaths and nutrition scientists, that such aliments should likewise be an important factor in its prevention?

But what are the facts as matters stand at present? It is significant that at a press conference (1966) it emerged that more than five million people in Britain were suffering from malnutrition, not all necessarily because of poverty, but because the public in general is unenlightened as regards food-values. One eminent doctor referred to the great number of old, solitary folk who tend to live almost entirely on tea, white bread-and-butter and white-sugared jam; meals lamentably deficient in both vitamins and mineral salts. Further, a report revealed that among the under-nourished were army recruits, miners, steel workers and other workers—also children; hence the prevalence of rickets.

But it would needlessly enlarge this book to expatiate on that deplorably high incidence of ordinary malnutrition. What chiefly concerns us here is the much less obvious form of it resulting from the omission to include in the daily diet enough of those natural unprocessed aliments, in naturopathic and biochemic literature listed under the headings of potassium foods and iron foods respectively, though some of them contain both minerals, and several others besides.

Potassium Foods

Especially rich in that particular cell-salt are *tomatoes*. And comparatively so are the following; lettuces, dandelion leaves (good in salads), celery, turnips, cabbages, etc., etc., whilst in fruits the highest content is in lemons, but it is also present in adequate quantities in peaches, apricots, grapes, oranges and cherries, also in several other fruits.

Iron Foods

These in particular are *spinach,* asparagus, lentils, radishes, onions, lettuce, leeks, all dark berries, strawberries; and of course cereals, wheat, rye, barley and oats. Many more of such natural aliments could be added.

The importance of iron may be gauged from what (the late) Dr. C. Stirling Saunders wrote in his *Guide To Biochemic Treatment,* viz. "that Iron (ferrum) gives warmth and magnetism to the body. It makes the blood red and the brain active... Iron causes hydrogen to be taken into the system through the lungs and thus breaks up fevers... People who lack Iron are irritable, lack self-control and poise..."

Of Potassium (Kali) he had even more to affirm. Briefly to quote: "Potassium is the builder and healer of the body. It supplies material for the muscles, making them pliant and elastic... It is also a healing agent. Potassium attracts oxygen, giving life and energy to the mind and body. It often prevents infection and reduces pain...."

As to drinks; natural fruit wines and beverages such as cider, perry, mead, lemonade, and fruit drinks generally, as well as yeasted ginger-beer, are richer in potassium than is (according to Dr. Forbes Ross) the finest whisky which contains none at all; hence the one-time habit of some whisky drinkers of diluting it with potash water was instinctively a wise one. But unfortunately, since then, soda-water has become the more widely used and popular diluent.

The important part which an adequate consumption of natural undemineralised foods has contributed to the efficacy of the aforementioned treatments, I think will be obvious to the reader. Nevertheless the following facts cannot rightly be ignored.

The Evils of Food Refining

This process, the idea of which was originally conceived in America many decades ago as a means of making more money in the milling industry, has since then created the supposition that food-refinement means food-improvement despite what nutrition scientists and naturopaths maintain to the contrary, and have done for years. Even so, there is a large percentage of the population who eat vast quantities of bread made from refined flour under the delusion that it is "the staff of life," as it was at one time called. And although additives are nowadays used by way of fortifying the white loaf, they do not make up for its lack of roughage, so important to facilitate healthy elimination.

Nor is flour the only food which loses through refinement; the same must also be said about sugar. Whilst white cane sugar has been found to be acid-forming, raw cane sugar, especially in the form of crude black molasses (called blackstrap molasses in

U.S.A.) is a most health-promoting nutriment, containing as it does iron, copper and magnesium, also phosphoric acid and potassium, besides being a rich source of the vitamins of the B family. Further, it is an effective natural laxative, and does not weaken the intestines as some laxatives tend to do. That it has any connection with cancer prevention may seem an unwarrantable assumption to cautious minded persons. Nevertheless a noteworthy fact is that workers on sugar plantations who are constantly sucking the crude sugar-cane, seldom if ever contract the disease.

Molasses can of course be taken in various ways according to individual tastes. It can be stirred into milk and then poured on to the breakfast cereals; it can be used as a substitute for white sugar to sweeten *café au lait*; or it may be diluted in hot water—two-thirds of a cupful to one teaspoonful of molasses, and taken as a drink at any convenient time of the day: better twice or thrice in the case of people so placed that they have to live for the most part on processed and hence de-natured aliments. (It may be mentioned that persons who find molasses too sickly as a drink, can add a little pure lemon juice to it without adversely affecting its valuable properties.) As farmers will know, for many years molasses have been used in making silage for cattle. But regarding its value as a health-giving substance for the consumption of humans, this has only in comparatively recent years to some extent come to be appreciated—and needless to say, especially by those numerous persons who in consequence of taking it have noticed a marked improvement in their health.

And now in this connection yet another natural aliment should certainly be mentioned.

Honey: A Perfect Food and Polychrest

The multiple virtues of this delectable "elixir of the gods" receive only little attention in orthodox medical textbooks; and thus many doctors of today are either unacquainted with its revealing history, or else are reluctant to prescribe so homely and simple a substance in the treatment of ills for which it has proved to be so curative.

Nor have scientific reasons for its power to cure been lacking. To the contrary, extensive investigations have shown genuine honey to be rich in vitamins and those mineral salts essential for the maintenance of sound health. It is also a potent bactericide, it feeds and stimulates the heart and other muscles, is remedial for digestive troubles because it does not ferment in the stomach; in short it is a natural energy-giving substance of the highest grade.

But of course not all types of honey are of equal quality. Indeed, as Dr. B. F. Beck, M.D. and Dorée Smedley pointed out in their comprehensive book *Honey and Your Health,* which is a mine of information; the properties of honeys vary according to the chemical characteristics of the nectar and pollen of the plants from which they are collected. These same authors also pointed out that honey could have a wider and better use in modern medical practice if studies were instituted to determine the types thereof best suited to particular ailments, either for cure or prevention. Whether or not the implication here is that an adequate intake of the right sort of honey could even prevent cancer, there is in any case this to be said; it is almost unheard of for a beekeper to get cancer. Furthermore, already centuries ago, honey had gained the reputation of being a life prolonger of quite phenomenal power (see Pliny's *Natural History,* 7th vol.). This reputation was founded on what the tax records revealed regarding the striking number of people who had lived to very great ages in areas where beekeeping was a major industry: those ages ranged from a hundred, and a few to even a hundred and thirty-five.

Nor is the conduciveness of honey to extreme longevity solely based on ancient observations hailing from foreign lands. In our own land, Britain, a study of parish registers and tombstones in old graveyards revealed records of a number of individuals who in the sixteenth and seventeenth centuries had died at ages ranging from one hundred and twenty-four to one hundred and fifty years. In all these cases honey had been an important ingredient in the daily diet.... It seems needless to add that mortals with incipient cancer in their blood could not have lived to such phenomenal ages.

The aforementioned list of treatments is not a complete one. Others there are about which it is too early to form any decisive conclusion, whilst some others are of a nature which cannot suitably be dealt with in this book. Suffice it in fairness to say that cancer-afflicted persons have been cured by entirely non-material methods; i.e. by prayer, magnetic healers, and Christian Science practitioners, in short by methods unrecognised by the orthodox profession. And although naturally there have been failures, the failures do not nullify those successes.

PART IV

PREVENTION: PRACTICAL SUGGESTIONS

Some Final Reflections

In view of the various means by which cancer has been cured, it is only reasonable to conclude that with some appropriate modifications it can be prevented; a matter which lies largely in the hands of the individual—the important thing, as the evidence goes to prove, being for him or her to include in the daily diet a sufficiency of those vital foods previously listed.

Nevertheless, though this advice which the nutrition scientists give out in their books and articles is sound the fact unfortunately cannot be denied that thousands of people are so situated that they are unable to observe these diatetic rules even if they wanted to.

There is, however, an alternative nowadays of which people could avail themselves; *viz.* the biochemic tablets *Kali phos.*, previously mentioned and obtainable from well stocked Health Food Stores. Apart from its other therapeutical value, this form of potassium, according to expert biotherapists may be regarded as the most essential preventive of cancer. It is not a drug nor a poison nor just a palliative, but a natural food for the cells and tissues.

As Dr. G. W. Carey, M.D., wrote in his large and learned book *The Biochemic System of Medicine* (published U.S.A.), "Kali Phos. is one of the most wonderful curative agents ever discovered by man, and the blessings it has already conferred on the race are many."

Those blessings, be it here explained, include the health-producing effects which *kali phos*. has on the brain and nerves: and if one agrees that in some cases, cancer may be caused by the too rapid depletion of potassium brought about by worry (Dr. Forbes Ross), then this particular cell salt, readily assimilated in its biochemic form, is wisely to be considered as a preventive. And certainly it would be also wise to consider it after some sufferer has undergone an operation. For, we repeat and emphasise here, that however adroitly a surgeon may extirpate a growth, its actual cause is not thereby removed from the body. And unless the patient afterwards takes or is treated by the preventive salt, there is no certainty that another growth may not subsequently develop.

Still—the reader must not suppose that there is only one way of supplying the body with potassium, seeing that Dr. Forbes Ross himself gave more than one method of doing this; the simplest for prevention being:

60 grains of bicarbonate or citrate of potash in a tumblerful of hot water that has been well boiled. To be drunk first thing in the morning, at least an hour before eating, or if inconvenient then, between meals. (One small level teaspoonful of pot. bic. equals approx. 60 grains.)

For those people, however, who may find it too irksome to follow these directions, the simplest way would be to pour and stir the level teaspoonful of the potash powder into some longish drink, say tea, or lemonade, orangeade or the like—it does not matter whether the drink be a hot or a cold one—and to make a regular habit of taking it once a day. But in the case of individuals who worry much, or have acquired a fear of the disease as a result, maybe, of frightening propaganda, then to take it twice a day (the first dose 60 grains, the second dose about half that amount) might be a wise rule to follow.

Lastly, considering those effective cancer-therapies which have existed for a number of years, the belief on the part of the public that cancer is a disease of an entirely mysterious nature, is one which would seem to require at least some modification. Granted there still remains a certain element of mystery concerning its actual manifestations, for which scientific research may someday provide a satisfactory explanation: meanwhile there is no explanation of the perhaps greater mystery as to why some people whose habits and general mode of life are entirely at variance with the commonly accepted laws of health, nevertheless remain free from that particular disease, whilst others with like habits and a similar life-pattern, unhappily for themselves, do not.

Nor in this digest of the various and varied theories, pronouncements and opinions regarding cancer, have I myself presumed to be able to explain that mystery. But if I have succeeded in adding any useful information to this brain-harassing subject, I shall consider my effort well rewarded.

Afterthought

In the domain of therapeutics the outlook is so constantly changing, that ever since I thought to have finished this book, there is something to be added about the position as it appears to stand today.

We live at a time when not only have many of our

purchased foods been sprayed with pesticides, and others grossly oversalted, but even *fluoride of sodium* (a deadly rat poison, very different from *fluoride of calcium*) is put into some of our water systems, despite the fact that already in 1958, the Association of American Physicians and Surgeons, with a membership of 15,000, passed a resolution strongly condemning it, and a leading authority on the subject summed it up as "the biggest piece of skulduggery ever put over on the American people."

These are strong words. But this condemnation has since come to be shared by many doctors in other countries beside U.S.A.; their reason being that they now know that some people are allergic to this artificially and poisonously fluoridised water.

With regard to the pesticides and chemical fertilizers now in use; granted that on this over-populated globe, such things have become a regrettable necessity. Yet latterly some cases have come to light of acute gastritis directly due to poisoning from insufficiently washed lettuces which had been chemically sprayed. Such cases might be somewhat exceptional, but are nevertheless significant, in that they go to disprove the notion that these said-to-be-safe sprayings are invariably harmless to man. In fact a grave suspicion has recently been mooted that the biologically active agents in widespread and indiscriminate use relative to food production may, in an accumulative though subtle way, be very adversely affecting the peoples of the world in the present epoch. One cannot take lightly this belief expressed by so eminent a histologist as Professor E. N. Willmer, F.R.S., of Cambridge University, in his impressive article* to that effect, and

* *The Observer*, August 20, 1967.

wherein he makes the warning suggestion that more restraint should be exercised in the use of the afore-mentioned substances. (Certainly greater care should be taken to wash thoroughly any foodstuffs thus sprayed.)

In fine: seeing that for years twentieth century man has been increasingly diverging from nature, and since we can no longer be certain that wise nutritional habits will nowadays suffice to keep the body-cells in that state of normalcy which is the surest protection against their becoming malignant, it seems only sensible to take advantage of one or other of those prophylactics referred to in this digest.